THE WELLNESS LIFESTYLE:

Achieving Health and Happiness on Your Own Terms.

Brenda B. Ortiz

Table of contents

Chapter 1: Introduction to Health and Wellness

Health and wellness are terms that are often used interchangeably, but they refer to two distinct concepts. Health refers to the state of being free from illness or injury, whereas wellness is a broader concept that encompasses physical, mental, and emotional well-being.

Physical health is often the first aspect of wellness that comes to mind, as it pertains to the body's ability to function properly. This includes factors such as fitness, nutrition, and sleep. Mental health, on the other hand, refers to our emotional and psychological well-being, encompassing our ability to cope with stress, maintain healthy relationships, and feel positive about ourselves.

Emotional well-being relates to our ability to manage our emotions and cope with the ups and downs of life. This includes feeling fulfilled, having a sense of purpose, and having positive social connections. Spiritual wellness relates to our sense of meaning and purpose in life and may involve practices such as meditation or prayer.

Overall, wellness is a holistic approach to health that recognizes the interdependence of various aspects of our lives. It involves striving to achieve a balance between different dimensions of well-being, and making choices that support our physical, mental, and emotional health.

Taking care of oneself is essential for living a healthy, happy, and fulfilling life. It involves making intentional decisions and engaging in activities that promote physical, mental, and emotional well-being. Here are some reasons why taking care of oneself is important:

Physical Health: Taking care of oneself helps to maintain physical health by providing the body with the necessary nutrients, exercise, and rest it needs to function optimally. Good self-care practices, such as eating a balanced diet, getting enough sleep, and exercising regularly, can help to prevent or manage chronic health conditions like heart disease, diabetes, and obesity.

Mental Health: Self-care is also crucial for maintaining good mental health. Engaging in activities that promote relaxation, mindfulness, and stress management can help to reduce feelings of anxiety and depression. Self-care also involves setting healthy boundaries, practicing self-compassion, and seeking support when needed, which can help to boost self-esteem and confidence.

Productivity and Performance: Taking care of oneself can improve productivity and performance in all areas of life. When we are well-rested, well-fed, and mentally and emotionally balanced, we are better able to focus, make decisions, and manage our time effectively. This can lead to better performance at work or school and more fulfilling relationships with family and friends.

Prevention of Burnout: Taking care of oneself can prevent burnout, which is a state of physical, mental, and emotional exhaustion that results from prolonged stress. Burnout can lead to feelings of disillusionment, cynicism, and decreased motivation. Engaging in self-care practices can help to prevent burnout by promoting relaxation, balance, and a sense of purpose.

In conclusion, taking care of oneself is crucial for living a healthy, happy, and fulfilling life. It can help to prevent chronic health conditions, improve mental health, increase productivity and performance, and prevent burnout. By making self-care a priority, individuals can enhance their overall quality of life and well-being

In today's fast-paced world, maintaining our health and wellness has become more challenging than ever before. We live in a society that glorifies busy schedules, unhealthy eating habits, and a sedentary lifestyle. However, the truth is that our health and wellness are the foundations upon which our lives are built. Without them, we cannot fully enjoy all that life has to offer. This is why it is so important to prioritize our health and wellness and to make them a central part of our daily lives.

In this book on health and wellness, we will explore the many different factors that contribute to our overall well-being. We will look at the importance of physical activity and a healthy diet, as well as the role that sleep, stress management, and mental health play in maintaining our overall health. We will also examine some of the most common health concerns facing people today, including obesity, diabetes, heart disease, and cancer, and explore strategies for preventing and managing these conditions.

Throughout this book, we will emphasize the importance of taking a holistic approach to health and wellness, recognizing that our physical, mental, and emotional well-being are all interconnected. We will provide practical tips and advice for making positive changes in our lives, and we will draw on the latest scientific research to support our recommendations.

Whether you are looking to improve your overall health and well-being or to address specific health concerns, this book is the perfect guide to help you achieve your goals. We hope that you will find this book both informative and inspiring, and that it will empower you to take control of your health and wellness, so that you can live your best life.

Chapter: 2 Nutrition

Nutrition refers to the study of the nutrients in food and how they are used by the body for growth, maintenance, and repair. It is the science of how the body utilizes nutrients from food to sustain life and prevent disease.

There are six essential nutrients that the body needs to function properly: carbohydrates, proteins, fats, vitamins, minerals, and water. Each of these nutrients serves a specific function in the body, and they must be consumed in appropriate amounts to maintain good health.

Carbohydrates are the primary source of energy for the body. They can be found in foods such as bread, pasta, rice, fruits, and vegetables. Proteins are important for building and repairing tissues and are found in foods like meat, fish, eggs, and beans. Fats also provide energy and help with the absorption of vitamins. They can be found in foods like oils, nuts, and dairy products.

Vitamins and minerals are important for the proper functioning of the body's systems. Vitamins are essential organic compounds that are needed in small amounts to maintain good health. They can be found in fruits, vegetables, and whole grains. Minerals are inorganic compounds that are also essential for good health. They can be found in foods like meat, dairy products, and leafy green vegetables.

Water is also essential for good health. It helps to regulate body temperature, transport nutrients and waste products, and lubricate joints. It is recommended that adults drink at least 8 glasses of water per day.

Eating a well-balanced diet that includes all of these nutrients is important for maintaining good health and preventing disease. In addition to consuming a healthy diet, regular physical activity and limiting the intake of unhealthy foods and beverages are also important for good nutrition.

Healthy Eating Habits

Healthy eating habits are practices that support overall health and well-being by providing the body with the nutrients it needs to function properly. Here are some examples of healthy eating habits you should inculcate:

Eat a variety of nutrient-rich foods: Include a variety of fruits, vegetables, whole grains, lean proteins, and healthy fats in your diet.

Control portion sizes: Pay attention to portion sizes and avoid overeating.

Limit processed and high-calorie foods: Avoid foods that are high in calories, saturated fat, trans fat, and added sugars.

Stay hydrated: Drink plenty of water and limit sugary drinks.

Eat mindfully: Take the time to savor your food and enjoy the experience of eating.

Plan ahead: Plan your meals and snacks in advance to avoid impulsive eating and unhealthy choices.

Listen to your body: Pay attention to your body's hunger and fullness cues, and eat when you're hungry and stop when you're full.

Cook at home: Cook your meals at home using healthy ingredients and cooking methods.

Eat slowly: Eat slowly and chew your food thoroughly to aid digestion and help you feel full.

Be flexible: Allow yourself to enjoy your favorite foods in moderation and make healthy choices most of the time.

Weight management strategies

There are many ways to manage weight and prevent diet-related diseases. Here are some strategies you can try:

Eat a healthy and balanced diet: Aim to eat a variety of nutrient-dense foods, such as fruits, vegetables, whole grains, lean proteins, and healthy fats. Avoid processed and high-calorie foods that are low in nutrients.

Control your portion sizes: Use smaller plates, bowls, and cups to help you eat less. Avoid eating in front of the TV or computer, which can lead to mindless eating.

Stay hydrated: Drink plenty of water throughout the day, as dehydration can sometimes be mistaken for hunger. Avoid sugary drinks, such as soda and fruit juice.

Exercise regularly: Aim for at least 150 minutes of moderate-intensity exercise each week. This can include activities like brisk walking, jogging, cycling, or swimming.

Get enough sleep: Aim for 7-8 hours of sleep per night, as lack of sleep can lead to overeating and weight gain.

Manage stress: Chronic stress can lead to overeating and weight gain. Find ways to manage stress, such as yoga, meditation, or deep breathing exercises.

Limit alcohol consumption: Drinking too much alcohol can lead to weight gain and increase your risk of developing chronic diseases.

Keep track of your progress: Use a food journal or app to track your food intake and exercise. This can help you stay accountable and make healthier choices.

Seek support: Enlist the help of friends, family, or a healthcare professional to support you in your weight loss and disease prevention efforts.

By adopting these strategies, you can manage your weight and reduce your risk of developing diet-related diseases

Chapter 3: Exercise and Fitness

Exercise and fitness are crucial components of a healthy lifestyle. Exercise refers to physical activity that is planned, structured, and repetitive for the purpose of improving or maintaining physical fitness. Fitness refers to the overall state of health and well-being, including cardiovascular health, muscle strength and endurance, flexibility, and body composition.

Regular exercise and physical activity can help prevent chronic diseases such as heart disease, diabetes, and obesity, and improve mental health and cognitive function. It can also improve sleep quality and boost energy levels. Some examples of exercise include aerobic activities such as running, cycling, and swimming, as well as resistance training such as weightlifting and bodyweight exercises.

It is important to find a form of exercise that is enjoyable and sustainable in the long term. It is also recommended to aim for at least 150 minutes of moderate-intensity exercise per week or 75 minutes of vigorous-intensity exercise per week, along with muscle-strengthening activities at least two days per week.

Before starting a new exercise program, it is important to consult with a healthcare professional to ensure it is safe and appropriate for your individual needs and health status.

The benefits of regular physical activity

Regular physical activity has numerous benefits for both physical and mental health. Here are some of the key benefits of regular physical activity:

- Improved cardiovascular health: Regular physical activity can help improve cardiovascular health by reducing the risk of heart disease, stroke, and high blood pressure.

- Better mental health: Regular physical activity can help improve mood, reduce symptoms of depression and anxiety, and improve overall mental health.

- Increased muscle strength and endurance: Regular exercise can help improve muscle strength and endurance, making it easier to perform daily activities and reducing the risk of injury.

- Improved flexibility and balance: Regular exercise can help improve flexibility and balance, reducing the risk of falls and injuries.

- Weight management: Regular physical activity can help manage weight by burning calories and building muscle mass.

- Reduced risk of chronic diseases: Regular physical activity can help reduce the risk of chronic diseases such as diabetes, osteoporosis, and certain types of cancer.

- Better sleep: Regular physical activity can help improve sleep quality and reduce the risk of sleep disorders.

- Increased energy levels: Regular exercise can help increase energy levels and reduce fatigue.

- Improved cognitive function: Regular physical activity has been shown to improve cognitive function and reduce the risk of cognitive decline in older adults.

Overall, regular physical activity is essential for maintaining good health and preventing chronic diseases. Even small amounts of exercise can have significant benefits, so it's important to find ways to incorporate physical activity into your daily routine.

Types of Exercise you can Engage

There are several different types of exercise that people can engage in to improve their physical fitness and overall health. Some of the most common types of exercise include:

- Aerobic exercise: Also known as cardio, this type of exercise increases your heart rate and breathing rate. Examples include running, cycling, swimming, and dancing.

- Strength training: This type of exercise focuses on building muscle mass and strength through resistance training, such as weight lifting, bodyweight exercises, and resistance bands.

- Flexibility exercises: These exercises are designed to improve your range of motion and prevent injury. Examples include stretching, yoga, and Pilates.

- Balance exercises: These exercises help improve your balance and stability, which can reduce your risk of falls and injuries. Examples include tai chi, yoga, and balance boards.

- High-intensity interval training (HIIT): This type of exercise involves alternating periods of high-intensity exercise with periods of rest or low-intensity exercise. It can be done with a variety of exercises, such as running, cycling, or bodyweight exercises.

- Low-impact exercises: These exercises are easier on the joints and are ideal for people with mobility issues or injuries. Examples include walking, swimming, and cycling.

- Functional training: This type of exercise focuses on movements that mimic everyday activities, such as lifting groceries or climbing stairs. Examples include squats, lunges, and push-ups.

- Sports-specific training: This type of exercise focuses on improving performance in a specific sport or activity, such as basketball, soccer, or martial arts.

It's important to choose a variety of exercises that you enjoy and that work for your fitness level and goals. A combination of different types of exercise can help you achieve optimal physical fitness and health.

How you can create an exercise plan
Creating an exercise plan can help you stay motivated and on track with your fitness goals. Here are some steps to help you create an exercise plan:

1. Set your goals: Determine what you want to achieve through exercise, such as improving your strength, losing weight, or

reducing stress. Make sure your goals are specific, measurable, and achievable.

2. Assess your current fitness level: Determine your current level of fitness by assessing your strength, flexibility, endurance, and other aspects of fitness. This will help you choose exercises that are appropriate for your fitness level.

3. Choose your exercises: Select exercises that are appropriate for your goals and fitness level. Choose a variety of exercises that target different muscle groups and aspects of fitness, such as strength training, cardio, flexibility, and balance.

4. Determine your frequency: Decide how often you want to exercise each week. Aim for at least 150 minutes of moderate-intensity aerobic exercise or 75 minutes of vigorous-intensity aerobic exercise per week, as well as two or more days of strength training per week.

5. Create a schedule: Create a schedule that includes the days and times you plan to exercise each week. Be realistic and choose times that work for your schedule.

6. Track your progress: Keep track of your progress by recording your workouts, such as the type of exercise, duration, and intensity. This can help you stay motivated and make adjustments to your plan as needed.

7. Make adjustments: Adjust your plan as needed based on your progress and any changes in your goals or fitness level. Be flexible and willing to make changes to your plan as needed.

Remember to consult with your healthcare provider before starting a new exercise plan, especially if you have any medical conditions or injuries.

How you can stay Motivated to your Exercise Plan

Creating an exercise plan and sticking to it can be challenging, but there are several steps you can take to help you stay motivated and committed. Here are some tips to help you create an exercise plan and stay motivated to it:

1. Set realistic goals: Be specific about what you want to achieve and set realistic goals. Whether it's weight loss, muscle gain, or improved fitness, make sure your goals are achievable and measurable.

2. Choose activities you enjoy: If you don't enjoy your workouts, it will be harder to stick to them. Find activities that you enjoy and that fit your lifestyle. This could be anything from running to yoga to weightlifting.

3. Plan your workouts: Plan your workouts ahead of time and make them a priority in

your schedule. Treat them like any other appointment and stick to them.

4. Start slowly and gradually increase intensity: If you're just starting out, don't try to do too much too soon. Start with a few minutes of exercise each day and gradually increase the intensity and duration over time.

5. Mix it up: Avoid boredom by mixing up your workouts. Try new activities or switch up your routine every few weeks to keep things interesting.

6. Get a workout partner: Working out with a friend or family member can help keep you accountable and motivated.

7. Reward yourself: Set up a reward system for yourself for reaching your goals. This could be anything from buying yourself new workout gear to treating yourself to a massage.

8. Track your progress: Keep track of your progress and celebrate your achievements. Seeing progress can be a great motivator to keep going.

Remember, staying motivated to your exercise plan is about finding what works for you and staying consistent with it. Be patient with yourself and don't give up if you have a setback. Keep pushing yourself and you will see results.

Chapter 4: Mental Health

Mental health refers to our overall psychological well-being, including our ability to manage our emotions, thoughts, and behaviors in a healthy and productive way. It encompasses many different aspects of our lives, such as our relationships with others, our ability to handle stress and adversity, and our sense of purpose and meaning.

Good mental health is essential for leading a fulfilling life and is closely tied to our physical health, with both affecting each other. When someone experiences poor mental health, it can impact their ability to function in their daily life, including their work, relationships, and overall quality of life. Some common mental health disorders include anxiety, depression, bipolar disorder, schizophrenia, and eating disorders.

It's important to take care of our mental health by seeking support when needed, maintaining healthy habits such as exercise and a balanced diet, practicing relaxation techniques like meditation, and seeking professional help when necessary. Stigma and misconceptions surrounding mental health can make it difficult for people to seek help or talk about their struggles, but it's essential to prioritize mental health as part of overall well-being.

Tips on Stress Management

Stress management refers to the strategies and techniques individuals use to cope with and reduce the negative effects of stress. Stress can arise from various sources, including work, relationships, financial problems, health issues, and more. Some common stress management techniques include:

- Exercise: Regular physical activity, such as walking, running, swimming, or yoga, can help reduce stress and improve mood.

- Mindfulness and meditation: Mindfulness and meditation practices involve focusing on the present moment and can help calm the mind and reduce stress.

- Time management: Poor time management can lead to stress. By planning and prioritizing tasks, individuals can feel more in control of their time and reduce stress.

- Relaxation techniques: Techniques such as deep breathing, progressive muscle relaxation, and visualization can help calm the body and mind.

- Social support: Talking to friends and family members, or joining support groups can help individuals feel more connected and reduce feelings of stress and anxiety.

- Healthy lifestyle habits: Eating a healthy diet, getting enough sleep, and avoiding drugs and alcohol can help reduce stress and promote overall well-being.

It is important to note that stress management techniques may vary from person to person, and it may take time to find the right combination of techniques that work best for you. If you find that your stress levels are significantly impacting your daily life, it may be helpful to seek support from a mental health professional.

Managing Anxiety & Depression.

Anxiety and depression can be difficult to deal with, but there are strategies that can help you manage and overcome these conditions. Here are some tips that may be helpful:

- Seek professional help: It's important to seek help from a mental health professional, such as a therapist or psychiatrist. They can provide a diagnosis and create a treatment plan tailored to your needs.

- Practice self-care: Taking care of your physical and emotional needs is crucial. Make sure you get enough sleep, exercise regularly, eat a healthy diet, and practice relaxation techniques like meditation or yoga.

- Challenge negative thoughts: Negative thinking patterns can fuel anxiety and depression. Try to identify negative thoughts and replace them with positive ones. This may take time, but with practice, it can become easier.

- Connect with others: Social support is important for mental health. Try to connect with friends, family, or a support group. You may also want to consider online support groups.

- Set goals: Setting small, achievable goals can help boost your self-esteem and give you a sense of purpose. Start with simple goals like cleaning your room or taking a walk outside.

- Consider medication: In some cases, medication may be necessary to manage anxiety and depression. Talk to your doctor or psychiatrist about whether medication is right for you.

Remember, managing anxiety and depression is a process that takes time and effort. Be patient with yourself and don't be afraid to ask for help when you need it.

How to Improve emotional well-being.

Improving one's emotional well-being involves developing strategies that promote positive emotions and reduce negative ones. Here are some tips for improving emotional well-being:

- Practice mindfulness: Mindfulness involves paying attention to the present moment, without judgment. By practicing mindfulness, you can develop an awareness of your thoughts and emotions and learn to observe them without becoming overwhelmed by them.

- Engage in physical activity: Regular exercise can improve mood, reduce stress, and increase energy levels. Even a short walk or yoga session can have a positive impact on emotional well-being.

- Cultivate positive relationships: Social support is essential for emotional well-being. Connect with friends, family, or colleagues who uplift and inspire you. Join groups or organizations that share your interests.

- Practice gratitude: Take time each day to reflect on the things you are grateful for. This can be as simple as appreciating a beautiful sunset, a delicious meal, or a supportive friend.

- Develop healthy coping strategies: Life can be challenging, and it's essential to have healthy ways to cope with stress and difficult emotions. This can include activities like journaling, meditation, or talking to a therapist.

- Get enough sleep: Sleep is essential for emotional well-being. Getting enough quality sleep can improve mood, increase energy levels, and reduce stress.

- Limit exposure to negative media: The news and social media can be overwhelming and contribute to negative emotions. Try to limit your exposure to negative news or social media and focus on positive, uplifting content.

Note that improving emotional well-being is a process that takes time and effort. Be patient with yourself and continue to practice self-care and healthy habits.

Chapter 5: Sleep

Sleep is a natural physiological state of rest in which the body and mind become inactive, allowing for rest, restoration, and recovery. It is essential for maintaining good health and overall well-being.

During sleep, the body goes through several stages of sleep, including light sleep, deep sleep, and rapid eye movement (REM) sleep. Each stage serves a different function in the body, with REM sleep being particularly important for memory consolidation and brain function.

The amount of sleep an individual needs can vary depending on a variety of factors, including age, lifestyle, and health conditions. Generally, adults require between 7-9 hours of sleep each night, while children and teenagers may need more.

Lack of sleep or poor sleep quality can have a significant impact on an individual's physical and mental health, including increased risk of obesity, diabetes, heart disease, and depression. It is important to establish good sleep habits and to seek medical attention if sleep disturbances persist.

Importance of Sleep Importance

Sleep is crucial for the overall health and well-being of an individual. Here are some of the reasons why sleep is important:

- Restores the body: During sleep, the body works to repair and restore tissues, and replenish energy levels. Sleep is essential for the immune system, which uses this time to fight off infections and illnesses.

- Enhances brain function: Sleep is essential for cognitive function, memory consolidation, and learning. Lack of sleep can lead to impaired concentration, memory, and decision-making abilities.

- Improves mental health: Sleep plays a significant role in regulating emotions and managing stress. Sleep deprivation can contribute to mood swings, anxiety, and depression.

- Maintains a healthy weight: Lack of sleep can disrupt the balance of hormones that control appetite, leading to overeating and weight gain.

- Reduces the risk of chronic diseases: Sleep deprivation has been linked to a higher risk of chronic conditions such as obesity, diabetes, and cardiovascular disease.

Overall, getting enough high-quality sleep is crucial for maintaining physical and mental health, as well as overall well-being.

How you can create a sleep-friendly environment

Creating a sleep-friendly environment is essential for getting a good night's rest. Here are some tips to create a conducive sleep environment:

- Keep the room cool and quiet: The ideal temperature for sleep is between 60 and 67 degrees Fahrenheit. Use earplugs or white noise machines to block out any outside noise.

- Make sure the bed is comfortable: Invest in a good quality mattress, pillows, and bedding that provide adequate support and comfort.

- Limit screen time before bed: Avoid using electronic devices such as smartphones, tablets, or laptops before bedtime. The blue light emitted by these devices can disrupt your sleep cycle.

- Dim the lights: Use dimmer switches or low-wattage bulbs to create a relaxing ambiance in the bedroom.

- Remove distractions: Keep the bedroom clutter-free and remove any items that can cause distractions such as televisions, work-related items, or exercise equipment.

- Stick to a sleep schedule: Go to bed and wake up at the same time each day, including weekends. This helps regulate your body's natural sleep-wake cycle.

- Use calming scents: Lavender or chamomile scents can promote relaxation and help you fall asleep faster.

By creating a sleep-friendly environment, you can improve the quality of your sleep, reduce sleep disturbances, and wake up feeling refreshed and energized.

Healthy Sleep Habits.

Establishing healthy sleep habits is important for your overall health and well-being. Here are some tips for improving your sleep:

- Stick to a consistent sleep schedule: Go to bed and wake up at the same time every day, even on weekends. This helps regulate your body's natural sleep-wake cycle.

- Create a relaxing sleep environment: Make sure your bedroom is cool, quiet, and dark. Use comfortable pillows and mattresses, and consider using blackout curtains or a white noise machine if necessary.

- Limit screen time before bed: The blue light emitted by electronic devices can disrupt your sleep cycle. Avoid using phones, tablets, or laptops for at least an hour before bed.

- Avoid caffeine, nicotine, and alcohol:
  These substances can interfere with your
  sleep quality. Avoid drinking caffeinated
  beverages or smoking cigarettes at least 4
  hours before bedtime. While alcohol may
  help you fall asleep, it can disrupt your
  sleep later in the night.

- Practice relaxation techniques: Activities
  like yoga, meditation, or deep breathing
  exercises can help you relax and prepare
  for sleep.

- Exercise regularly: Regular exercise can
  improve sleep quality, but avoid
  exercising within 3 hours of bedtime.

- Stick to a pre-sleep routine: Develop a
  calming pre-sleep routine that signals to
  your body that it's time for sleep. This
  could include reading a book, taking a
  warm bath, or listening to relaxing music.

By incorporating these habits into your daily routine, you can establish healthy sleep habits and improve your overall sleep quality.

Chapter 6: Relationships and Social Support

Relationships and social support are important aspects of human well-being and can significantly impact our mental and physical health.

Healthy relationships, whether romantic, familial, or platonic, provide a sense of belonging, love, and support. They offer a safe space for individuals to express themselves and share their emotions, thoughts, and experiences. These relationships can also provide a sense of purpose and meaning, helping individuals to navigate life's challenges.

Social support, or the assistance and comfort provided by family, friends, and community, can also have a significant impact on our well-being.

It can provide emotional support, such as empathy and understanding, as well as tangible assistance, such as financial or practical help. Social support can also act as a buffer against stress and help individuals cope with difficult situations.

On the other hand, negative relationships and lack of social support can have detrimental effects on mental and physical health. Social isolation and loneliness, for example, have been linked to an increased risk of depression, anxiety, and other mental health problems. Poor relationships, such as those characterized by conflict, abuse, or neglect, can also lead to negative health outcomes and increase the risk of chronic disease.

Overall, fostering healthy relationships and seeking out social support can have numerous benefits for our well-being. It's important to prioritize these aspects of our lives and seek help if we are struggling to build or maintain positive relationships and support systems.

The importance of healthy relationships

Healthy relationships are incredibly important for our well-being in a variety of ways. Here are some of the key reasons why:

- Emotional support: Healthy relationships provide us with emotional support and a sense of belonging. They give us a space to express our feelings and receive empathy and validation from others. This support can help us cope with stress, anxiety, and other difficult emotions.

- Improved mental health: Strong relationships have been linked to improved mental health outcomes, such as reduced rates of depression and anxiety. Having someone to talk to and share our problems with can help us feel less alone and overwhelmed.

- Physical health benefits: Positive relationships have also been linked to

improved physical health outcomes, such
as lower blood pressure and reduced risk
of chronic illness. This may be due in part
to the stress-reducing effects of social
support.

- Increased self-esteem: Being in a healthy
  relationship can help us feel more
  confident and secure in ourselves.
  Knowing that someone cares about us and
  values our opinions can boost our
  self-esteem and sense of self-worth.

- Personal growth: Healthy relationships
  can provide opportunities for personal
  growth and learning. They can challenge
  us to become better communicators,
  listeners, and problem-solvers, and help us
  develop greater empathy and
  understanding of others.

Overall, healthy relationships are essential for
our well-being and can have far-reaching
benefits for both our mental and physical health.

It's important to prioritize building and
maintaining positive relationships in our lives.

How you can build and maintain social connections

Building and maintaining social connections can be important for our overall well-being and happiness. Here are some tips for building and maintaining social connections:

- Be open and friendly: Be approachable and open to meeting new people. Smile and make eye contact with others, and engage in small talk to start building connections.

- Join groups and organizations: Joining groups or organizations that align with your interests can be a great way to meet new people and build social connections. Consider joining a sports team, book club, or volunteer organization.

- Attend social events: Attend social events, such as parties or networking events, where you can meet new people and build connections. If you are nervous about attending events alone, invite a friend to join you.

- Keep in touch with friends and family: Regularly check in with friends and family members to maintain your relationships. Use social media, text messages, or phone calls to stay connected.

- Show interest in others: When you meet new people, ask questions and show interest in their lives. People often enjoy talking about themselves, and showing interest can help build a connection.

- Make time for social activities: Make socializing a priority by scheduling regular social activities with friends and family. This could include going out for dinner, taking a class together, or planning a weekend getaway.

- Be reliable and dependable: Be a reliable
  friend by keeping your commitments and
  being there for others when they need you.

Building and maintaining social connections
takes effort and time. Don't be discouraged if it
takes time to build strong connections. Keep at
it, and you will likely see positive results over
time.

How you can manage conflict

Conflict is a natural part of life, and it can arise
in any setting, whether it's personal or
professional. Managing conflict is an important
skill that can help you maintain healthy
relationships, improve communication, and
achieve your goals. Here are some steps to
effectively manage conflict:

- Stay calm: Try to remain calm and
  composed when conflict arises. Avoid
  getting defensive or aggressive, as this can
  escalate the situation. Take a deep breath

and try to approach the situation with a level head.

- Listen: Listen actively to the other person's point of view. Try to understand their perspective and show empathy. Let them express themselves fully without interruption.

- Communicate: Express your own thoughts and feelings in a respectful manner. Use "I" statements instead of "you" statements to avoid sounding accusatory. Try to be specific and clear about what you want to communicate.

- Find common ground: Look for areas of agreement and common ground. Focus on shared goals or interests that you both care about.

- Explore solutions: Brainstorm possible solutions together. Be open to compromise and be willing to find a solution that works for both parties.

- Agree on a course of action: Once you have identified a solution, agree on a course of action. Be clear about what each party needs to do to implement the solution.

- Follow up: Check in later to see how the solution is working. If it's not working, revisit the issue and try to find another solution together.

Conflict can be an opportunity for growth and improvement in relationships. By managing conflict effectively, you can strengthen relationships and create a more positive and productive environment.

Chapter 7: Preventive Health

Preventive health refers to actions and practices that aim to prevent the occurrence or development of illnesses or diseases. These actions can be taken by individuals, healthcare providers, or public health organizations to promote and maintain overall health and wellbeing. Some common examples of preventive health measures include:

- Regular medical checkups and screenings: These can help identify potential health issues early on, making them easier to treat.

- Vaccinations: Immunizations can prevent a wide range of diseases, including measles, polio, and the flu.

- Healthy lifestyle habits: Eating a balanced diet, getting regular exercise, avoiding smoking and excessive alcohol consumption, and managing stress can all contribute to good health and reduce the risk of chronic diseases.

- Environmental controls: Taking measures to reduce exposure to harmful substances in the environment, such as air pollution or toxic chemicals, can also promote good health.

- Education and awareness: Public health campaigns and education programs can help people understand the importance of preventive health measures and encourage them to take action to protect their health.

Preventive health is an important aspect of healthcare, as it can help reduce the overall burden of disease and improve quality of life for individuals and communities.

The importance of preventive health measures

Preventive health measures are important because they can help individuals maintain good health and prevent the onset of many diseases and conditions. Some of the key benefits of preventive health measures include:

- Early detection of diseases: Regular screenings and check-ups can help detect diseases and conditions in their early stages when they are most treatable.

- Reduction in healthcare costs: Preventive measures can help reduce the need for expensive medical procedures and treatments, thereby lowering healthcare costs.

- Improved quality of life: By taking steps to prevent illness, individuals can improve their overall quality of life and avoid the

pain, discomfort, and disability associated
with many chronic conditions.

- Increased lifespan: Preventive health
  measures can help individuals live longer,
  healthier lives by reducing the risk of
  serious illnesses.

- Public health benefits: Preventive
  measures can also help prevent the spread
  of infectious diseases and protect public
  health.

Chapter 8: Alternative and Complementary Medicine

Alternative and complementary medicine refers to practices and therapies that are not considered mainstream or conventional medical treatments. These practices and therapies may be used in conjunction with, or instead of, conventional medical treatments.

Some examples of alternative and complementary medicine practices and therapies include:

- Acupuncture: A practice originating in traditional Chinese medicine that involves the insertion of needles into specific points on the body to promote healing and alleviate pain.

- Chiropractic care: A form of manual therapy that involves manipulation of the

spine and other joints to improve function
and alleviate pain.

- Herbal medicine: The use of herbs and
plant-based remedies for therapeutic
purposes.

- Homeopathy: A system of alternative
medicine based on the concept that "like
cures like," in which extremely diluted
substances are used to stimulate the body's
natural healing processes.

- Naturopathic medicine: A system of
alternative medicine that uses natural
remedies and therapies to promote healing
and prevent disease.

- Mind-body therapies: Practices that focus
on the connection between the mind and
body, such as meditation, yoga, and tai
chi.

- Ayurveda: A system of traditional medicine that originated in India that uses a combination of herbs, diet, exercise, and lifestyle practices to promote health and well-being

While some alternative and complementary medicine practices have been shown to be effective for certain conditions, others have not been scientifically validated or may even be harmful. It is important to approach these therapies with caution and to discuss their use with a qualified healthcare provider. Additionally, it is important to remember that alternative and complementary medicine should not be used as a substitute for conventional medical treatments for serious or life-threatening conditions.

Benefits and risks of alternative and complementary medicine

While there are several benefits associated with CAM, there are also risks that should be considered.

Benefits of CAM:

- Holistic Approach: CAM therapies focus on the whole person, including their physical, emotional, and spiritual well-being. This holistic approach can lead to greater overall health and wellness.

- Fewer Side Effects: CAM therapies often have fewer side effects than conventional treatments. For example, acupuncture does not involve any medication and therefore does not have the same risks associated with medication use.

- Greater Control Over Health: CAM therapies often allow individuals to take a more active role in their own health and wellness. By choosing therapies that work best for them, they can feel empowered and in control of their health.

- Potential for Complementary Benefits: CAM therapies can sometimes complement conventional treatments. For example, a patient with cancer may use acupuncture to manage nausea and pain while undergoing chemotherapy.

Risks of CAM

- Lack of Scientific Evidence: Many CAM therapies lack rigorous scientific evidence to support their effectiveness. This can be concerning, especially when patients forego conventional treatments in favor of CAM therapies.

- Interaction with Conventional Treatments: Some CAM therapies can interact with conventional treatments, which can be dangerous. For example, herbal supplements can interact with prescription medications and cause adverse effects.

- Delayed or Inadequate Treatment: Choosing CAM therapies over conventional treatments can sometimes delay or prevent adequate treatment for serious conditions. This can have serious consequences for an individual's health.

- False Claims: The lack of regulation in the CAM industry can lead to false claims and ineffective treatments being marketed to vulnerable individuals.

In summary, CAM therapies can provide a range of benefits, including a holistic approach to health, fewer side effects, greater control over health, and potential complementary benefits. However, there are also risks associated with CAM, including a lack of scientific evidence, interaction with conventional treatments, delayed or inadequate treatment, and false claims. It is important for individuals to carefully weigh the benefits and risks of CAM and consult with a healthcare provider before making any decisions about their healthcare.

Integrating CAM in your Lifestyle.

Integrating alternative and complementary medicine into a healthy lifestyle involves understanding both the benefits and risks associated with these practices. Here are some steps to help you do so:

- Research the alternative and complementary medicine practices you are considering: Before incorporating any new practice into your health routine, it is important to do your research. Look for reliable sources of information, such as medical journals or reputable websites, to learn about the benefits and risks associated with the practice.

- Consult with a healthcare professional:
  Talk to a healthcare professional, such as a
  naturopathic doctor or integrative
  medicine practitioner, who has experience
  with alternative and complementary
  medicine. They can help you evaluate the
  potential benefits and risks, as well as
  recommend safe and effective practices.

- Consider your personal health history and
  current health status: It is important to
  consider your individual health needs
  when deciding whether to incorporate
  alternative and complementary medicine
  practices into your lifestyle. For example,
  if you have a pre-existing medical
  condition or are taking prescription
  medication, some practices may not be
  suitable for you.

- Start slowly and track your progress: If
  you decide to try a new practice, start
  slowly and keep track of how it affects
  you. This can help you identify any

positive or negative effects and adjust your approach accordingly.

- Focus on whole-body health: Rather than relying solely on alternative and complementary medicine practices, it is important to focus on whole-body health. This includes getting regular exercise, eating a healthy diet, managing stress, and getting enough sleep.

Overall, integrating alternative and complementary medicine practices into a healthy lifestyle can provide a range of benefits, but it is important to approach these practices with a balanced and informed perspective. By doing your research, consulting with healthcare professionals, and focusing on whole-body health, you can create a safe and effective health routine that works for you.

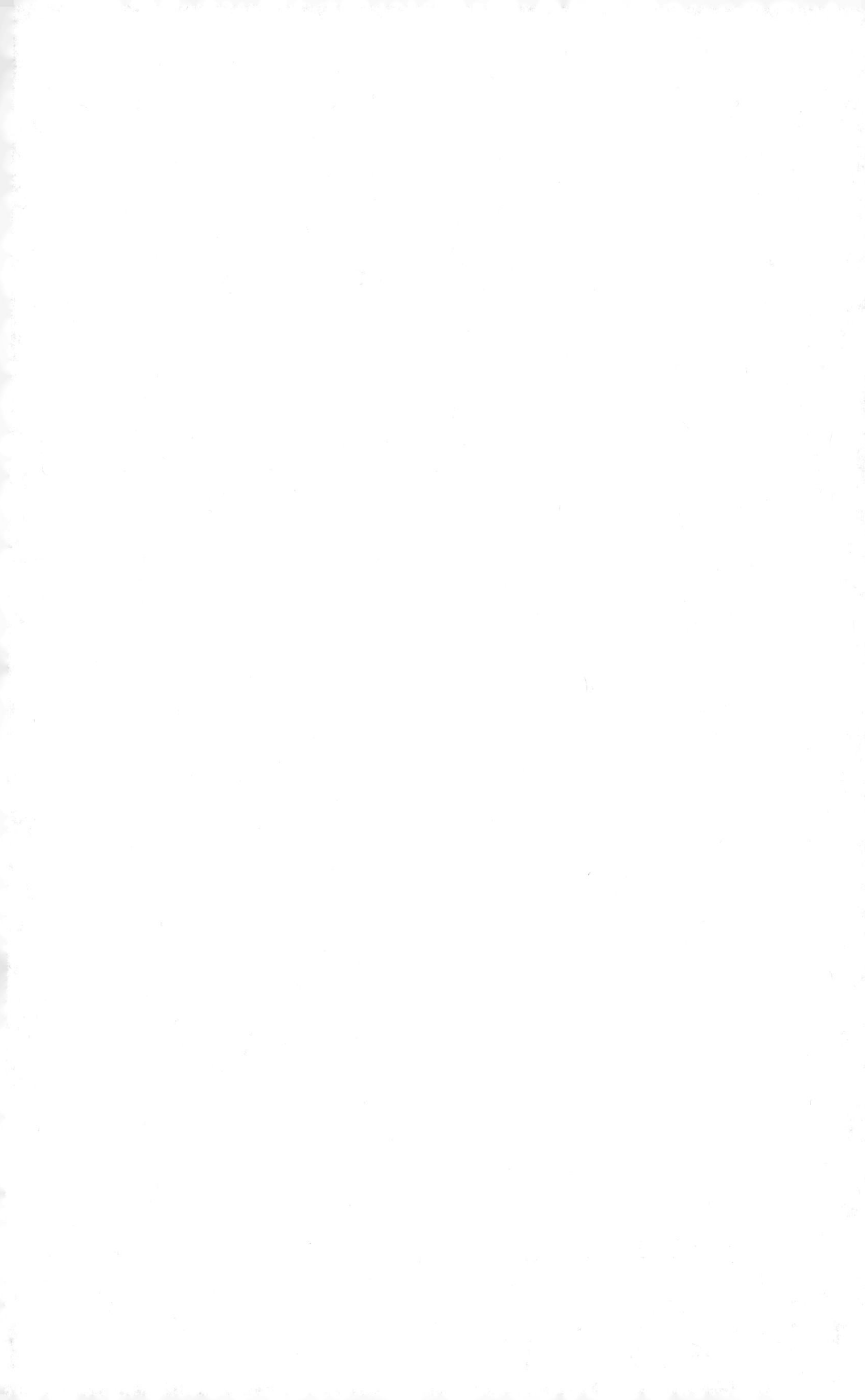